Potty Tr

Chairs

#1 Parenting Guide for Choosing a

Perfect Potty Chair

Regina Williams

ISBN: 978-1-63750-253-2

Table of Contents

Introduction

There are various potty chairs that may be purchased when you start potty training your kid. However, all of them are very different and also have cool features too.

It could be hard to determine which one to buy and which one is best for your son or daughter. However, this is an essential aspect of toilet training, for your child must be comfortable and feel secure when it pertains to toilet training, and the toilet chair makes this happen.

Your kids have to be capable of getting to the toilet easily and also go directly to the toilet easily. The simpler it is to allow them to go directly to the toilet, the much more likely they'll want to use the toilet. Additionally, it is fun to use the toilet because they have a toilet seat that they like to go to, such as a musical one or one with common characters on it, and this will motivate them as well to use the toilet.

We understand why and also have created this book on toilet chairs and everything that you'll require to learn about them too, and that means you can pick the one which is most beneficial for your son or daughter. You can look over here to see the actual differences between all of them to make choosing one so easy, after a much better potential for choosing the one your child prefers.

Chapter 1

What to Know about Choosing a Potty Chair or Potty Seat

What is the difference?

Why use one or the other for toilet training.

The difference between a Potty Seat and Potty Chair initially appear to be a simple question to answer. In most cases, the variations are a little more included. Our primary concentration is to offer you enough quality information to help you make the best decision for your loved ones.

You must take a number of different aspects to choose which is the best fit for your loved ones. Additionally, you may be thinking about; "Why must I use one with the other"? A way to answer this is to;

- *Know what your son or daughter needs.*

- *Know what your son or daughter likes.*

This truly is dependent upon a number of different aspects such as; exactly what will work best for your loved ones and what your requirements, needs and wants are?

What may be right for just one family doesn't invariably imply that it is right for yours; truthfully, this is dependent upon your family's needs and desires.

Following this discussion, you might come to the final outcome that both can be hugely helpful tools to work with you in potty training your kid. The easiest explanation of both would be that the potty chair is a standalone product that is totally independent on a toilet and a potty seat is a stationary addition to your existing toilet seat or can replace it altogether and can grow with your son or daughter.

There are benefits and drawbacks concerning all sorts of product that is in the marketplace. We cover most of them to work with you to make the best decision for your loved ones.

First, we will uncover the professionals, the cons and shall cover a lot of the aspects regarding the toilet chair. Toilet Seats are portable, most of them are light-weight enough for your son or daughter to have the ability to move it himself or herself. Also, toilet Chairs can be found with tempting and fun sizes and shapes, some with musical features.

Fun character types and designs can adorn the toilet seat. This can be considered a highly motivating aspect to your child; wonderful designs can be visually motivating to your child and this can be an important aspect to consider, for children of this age have a tendency to learn more effectively when they are visually stimulated.

So, if your son or daughter is enthralled with pets or a favorite personality, viewing this on the seat may be the extra drive that your son or daughter needs to deal with this next thing in their development.

A few of these seats are multipurpose, such as our throne themed chair that are ideal for you little prince or princess coordinating into nearly every décor. These toilet seats can be changed into a rocking seat for your son or daughter to use once once they outgrow this level of development.

A few of these wooden toilet chairs feature a wall paper

and publication holder that may be removed as well.

Potty Seats are child size that allows their little feet to have the ability to reach the ground, which shall encourage a far more natural toilet position that will aid them in producing a highly effective elimination of their waste materials.

Potty Seats promotes independency. At this time of development, children have a tendency to test their limitations while craving to be relatively impartial, which when utilizing a toilet chair, they don't really have to require assistance.

Chapter 2

Types of Toilet Chairs

Let your son or daughter choose the toilet training chair or seats they need; there are many that are extremely playful and fun and it might be the incentive your son or daughter must want to have.

With regards to toilet training, ensuring children have all the correct equipment to visit is really important. They have to feel safe and sound while heading, as well as be comfortable and also access the toilet easily. The greater unpleasant and difficult it is to allow them to go, the more unlikely they'll want to.

Ensuring they have the right potty seat to use could possibly be the perfect incentive for the kid to figure out how to use the potty. Toilet chair come in a huge selection of colors, styles and functions for a kid to use.

Here's our wide selection of potty seats:

- toddler toilet chair.

- travel toilet chairs.

- wooden toilet chairs.

- musical toilet chairs.

- multifunctional potties.

- customized potty chairs.

All these can be purchased in a huge selection of styles and colors to choose from. The toddler toilet chairs are extremely fun and whimsical.

If your kid likes princesses or cars, animals or bright colors can be a fantastic choice. These come in chairs that are formed liked fun pets, as well as with abstract designs in shiny pinks and blues.

Chapter 3

How to choose the best potty Chair?

When on the seek out for the best toilet chair you would run into a variety of options, styles, designs and sizes. This consists of potty chair that are of one-piece designs or multifunctional toilet chairs that can be utilized for many reasons like travel toilet chair when touring with toddlers.

5 Key Different Potty Chair Variation:

- One Piece Toilet Chair.

- Removable Chamber.

- Multi-function Toilet Chairs.

- Potty chair.

- Travel Potty Chair & Seats.

One Piece Design

Pros:

- Simple and portable.

- Low profile – makes it possible for toddler to get on and off and encourages the greater natural squatting position for toileting.

- Light-weight and compact.

- Inexpensive.

- No pinching or sharp edges

Cons:

- Have to subject the entire toilet chair in the toilet.

- Due to low profile and light-weight, toddler may trip like when there is a toy on the floor.

- Too small for much larger children

Removable Chamber Chair

Pros:

- Makes tidy up easy.

- Some models include lids.

- Smaller version can be portable.

- It's a most common kind of potty chairs

Cons:

- Might lead to pinching of child's bottom level or thighs.

- Most model aren't very portable.

Multifunction Toilet Chairs

Pros:

- 2-in-1 Design offers not just a potty seat but a removable toilet seat.

- 3-in-1 Design offers a toilet chair, potty chair and step stool design.

- 4-in-1 Design offers toilet chair, potty chair, step stool and storage space compartments for playthings, books, and other rewards.

- Easy transitioning to mature toilet

Cons:

- Large and bulky.

- Not easily portable.

- Costlier than traditional toilet chairs.

- Limited designs.

Potty Chairs

Pros:

- No tidy up.

- Using the true potty

Cons:

- Toilet can be too much for some children - makes it hard to relax when feet are dangling.

- May hinder independence for child needs to be assisted.

- Must be removed for adult use.

Travel Toilet Chairs

Travel potty seats & travel toilet seats

Pros:

- Convenient.

- Security and child's comfort.

- Sanitary.

- Life saver! If you are out in the street you can't plan toilet breaks for small children.

Cons:

- Not created for every day use.

- Additional expense

C h a p t e r 4

Potty Trained in One Day- Exactly what does it mean?

Sounds great does it not?

Or is too good to be true?

It all boils down to perspective and anticipations.

This technique is not really a magic pill, but like everything in life, with planning, preparation and determination you can succeed in anything.

It will require work and energy on your part and yes, you will need to clean up toilet accidents. Most of us study from our errors so your child will never be any different.

It is however really a successful method that has successfully worked for most parents. The main one day is the "WEDDING DAY". This is actually the day when the real potty training is performed as well as your child gives up diapers permanently and begin using "big child" toilet training pants.

The Toilet Training Process

However, as other activities in life, you should be able to have an enjoyable and successful "WEDDING DAY" and this implies you spending time preparing and planning this day. The look and planning could take from one hour to some weeks depending about how ready you are as well as your child. The time spent before necessary the "WEDDING DAY" is really dependent upon your son or daughter. Some children do not require any follow-up, but others may.

So, what's Potty Training in One Day?

It is a successful method to toilet train your son or daughter; Your child gives up diapers upon this day and can figure out how to pee on the toilet, and can also learn what's expected of him/her so far as heading to the toilet is concerned.

You on the other hands; must expend time and energy before that day by getting all the merchandise collectively and then planning your son or daughter and yourself because of the day (you already are carrying this out by scanning this book). You will need to mentally and actually get ready to take care of toilet incidents and clean ups from these toilet accidents. Following the big day, you'll also have to completely clean up more toilet accidents and follow-up with your son or daughter and ensure that he or she is clear on what you anticipate from him or her.

A lot of people who opt for this technique are amazed by how quickly the youngster learns as the potty incidents becomes limited by a couple of days. Most children will be incident free in a single week; however, you have those that never have mishaps, and then you have those that will have incidents for two weeks.

Stay with it, as well as your child, and there will be incident free scenario in fourteen days or less!! Forget about diapers or pull-ups!!

Still skeptical? Read well on how this toilet training in one-day method has been working for other parents.

Chapter 5

Two Simple Ideas for Potty Training in One Day

The technique described in the Parent's Potty Training Guide: How exactly to Potty Train in a single Day is dependent on two simple concepts:

- The first concept is dependent on the actual fact that the ultimate way to learn something is to instruct it. We realize that children study from viewing and hearing. They learn actions and attitudes and can copy things they have seen. So, what's better than utilizing a doll to model the correct toilet training behavior for your son or daughter?

- The next concept is dependent on the actual fact

that behavior is shaped by consequence. Like a parent, you know that children study from the results of their actions and you almost certainly have previously used this as a highly effective parenting tool.

You will find that the two types of consequences to use are logical and natural. Natural results from the child's own activities. Logical results are also due to behavior, but it is imposed by the mother or father.

So, basically, with your assistance, your son or daughter will train a doll called Potty Scotty or Toilet Patty, an anatomically young toilet training doll specially made to toilet train the correct "going toilet" behaviors. Your son or daughter begins to learn that the natural outcome of consuming is the desire to urinate, and the reasonable effect of urinating in a toilet are rewards such as verbal &

nonverbal praise, treats, playthings and a good celebration toilet party.

Making Scotty go to the Toilet

Then, your son or daughter will train the doll the natural consequence of not using the potty, which is wet underwear. The reasonable consequence of the undesired behavior is training heading back and forth to the toilet.

It is as easy as that. And it works.

However, like the majority of things in life, success is a result of preparation and planning. There is absolutely no miracle pill, it will require some work and energy on your part to reach your goals.

My Parent's Toilet Training Guide explains how to steer your child detail by detail.

Chapter 6

Potty Chair and Toilet Seats

Although lots of commercial products can make life easier, the only must have item for toilet training is a toilet. In the past, a simple container or dish sufficed for everybody, however the added comfort and interesting colors of commercial brands enhance small children's motivation.

The two basic types of commercial potties are:

Potty Chair

They are self-contained models that take a seat on the floor. These are low enough to increase children's emotions of security, and increase a toddler's interest when they are alone. The drawback is that a detachable dish must be transported to the toilet emptied and rinsed after every use. Also, some children have a problem with the changeover from potty seat to the standard toilet.

Potty Seats

They are put on the seat of a normal toilet, developing a smaller space so children don't fall in. Some small children like the sensation to be developed that originates from using the toilet like old siblings and parents, however, many youngsters fear so much the elevation. Climbing up can be difficult, and a scary fall can complicate training.

Below are a few features to consider:

- Stability - The bottom of a toilet seat should be at least as wide at the very top for small children and wider at the bottom. This is the very best for babies.

- Splash Guards - Although splash guards are a benefit for sanitation by directing blast of urine, which is particularly useful for males, many tots finish up with an agonizing bump sooner or later, and won't want to visit near the toilet afterward. Climbing on a splash safeguard to log off the toilet chair can be difficult enough to result in a fall. Splash guards should be cushioned or detachable. Normally, make sure there can be an inch between your splash safeguard and the child's crotch.

- Security - Toilet seat should fasten to the toilet chair securely. Check the grips.

- Potty Dish - Bigger is way better for avoiding

spills. The dish should be easy enough to eliminate so that small children can vacant them independently.

- Chair - A chilly, hard potty chair is less inviting when compared to a soft one. Choose a model with a padded chair.

- Arm rests - If toilet seats have arm rests, children will automatically grab one and hold fast onto it as they sit back, which can cause the seat to overturn. Prevent them.

- Stepping stool - Some toilet chair convert to toilet seat, which can cut costs later on.

- Portability - Some toilet chairs collapse down for journeying. Make sure that the hinges are stuffy therefore the device won't collapse during normal use.

- Some children totally reject one toilet seat/chair, refusing even to look close to it, yet are extremely taken with another brand.

Chapter 7

Toilet Training and Travel

A big change in environment, the effect of a vacation or another travel is another common reason behind toilet-related problems amongst children.

Travel programs that require to take the kid from a familiar toilet or toilet, may create stress that then leads to mishaps or constipation.

Some responses are just short-term and disappear after the child gets used to the new schedule or has returned to the old one, some business lead to negative behavior, such as withholding stool or delaying urination that calls for weeks or a few months to correct.

In order to avoid such problems, you need to keep your

son or daughter's toilet experience whilst travelling as similar as possible to the routine he follows at home.

If you're vacationing by car, consider taking your son or daughter's toilet along, or you could have a travel potty.

When flying, take your son or daughter to the toilet at the airport terminal before you take the plane, and bring along familiar stuffed animals or other favorite items that could make public or hotel toilets less frightening.

Intend to accompany your son or daughter to the toilet and be prepared to encourage toilet use more than if you weren't traveling.

Chapter 8

Choosing an Ideal Potty

There are so many potties in the marketplace, how will you know which to choose? Prior to making your purchase, we've outlined the critical indicators to consider when deciding on a potty.

Is your son or daughter prepared to make the leap out of diapers? Congrats! Now you have the best purchase: the toilet. We've divided the key decisions and key features to consider what you look out for, the perfect toilet for your son or daughter as well as your toilet. If she's interested, take your child along on the shopping trip; if not, take your tot's measurements prior to you heading to the store. Below are a few things to retain in mind.

Plan for Storage space

You will find two main types of potties: a stand-alone potty and a seat reducer. When searching for a stand-alone toilet, consider three important features: security, size, and simplicity. The toilet seat must be steady, your toddler's bottom level must fit easily on the chair, and the toilet should be easy to use and easy to completely clean. A stand-alone toilet has lots of benefits for your tot; it's kid-size, which means that your child can get on and off by himself, and during prolonged periods of wanting to go, especially for number 2, your toddler will not be monopolizing the toilet (this is particularly important to consider for one-toilet households). Plus, keeping the standard toilet free enables you or a mature sibling demonstrate toilet skills at exactly the same time younger child is toilet training.

Chair reducers, which is used on a traditional toilet seat and decrease the band to an appropriate, kid-friendly size, likewise have specific benefits. They're less costly when compared to a stand-alone toilet and take up less living area. Your son or daughter gets used to the standard toilet, which helps prevent another changeover from stand-alone toilet to adult toilet, and there is certainly even less clutter (if anything) to completely clean after use. Plus, chair reducers can be considered a good fit for kids who prefer to duplicate. They can be considered a great motivator for kids who prefer to mimic their old siblings, cousins, or friends. But retain in brain that if you select a chair reducer, you may want to choose stool for it can help your child get right up on the toilet and provide sufficient foot support whenever a child is expelling pee or poop.

Most stand-alone potties and chair reducers also include handles, which can help your son or daughter feel better. They provide kids something to carry on with, which helps them drive. With chair reducers, handles provide a simple way to get the chair and put it away or suspend it for storage space. If you are still uncertain what your son or daughter will choose, choose a multitasking toilet that is capable of doing various functions and save space. Many stand-alone potties have detachable seats you can use as a chair reducer or toilet seat and shut lids that can dual as stools.

Consider Toilet Fit and Size

Potties come in a number of levels and rim sizes, so it is important to choose one with a good fit. In case your toddler's bottom level is draping on the chair or barely within the inside rim, he or she will probably feel unpleasant, stressed, or both," Crane says. The proper size chair will let your son or daughter's bottom level rest easily and solidly on the chair, with her feet firmly on to the floor or stool.

Search for Splash Guards

If you're toilet training a kid, you can lessen post-potty cleanup by choosing the chair with a splash safeguard. Choose one which is high enough to keep the pee in the toilet but isn't so high that it'll be difficult for your tot to sit back on the toilet by himself.

Consider Extra Fun Features

Potties can be found with a number of themes, lamps, songs, and sound files, but are they worthwhile? For some, this might boost your child's interest, particularly if your son or daughter was the one to choose the competition car flushing sound or the marvelous wand reward track toilet. But it's definitely not essential, Parenting Just like a Pro says, "A lot more than any light show, sticker, or little bit of candy, the matter that delights your son or daughter the most is your compliment. So, anticipate to clap the hands, give a large hug, or execute a special dance to celebrate your son or daughter's success, and miss the electronics."

Check Simple Emptying

In the event that you choose a stand-alone toilet, you should have more dirty work to do. Check the box's outside or online product critiques to observe how many steps must vacant and clean the container. Some are a straightforward, one or two step process; while others require that you disassemble half the toilet each and every time.

Chapter 9

Advantages and Disadvantages of Toilet Chair/Seat

Woow! It's time for you to potty train your child! Potty training will surely test thoroughly your patience but an appropriate potty will surely make the work easier.

There are a wide variety of potties on the marketplace that finding the right one can be considered a task alone. That's where this guide comes in; by the time you finish reading. you'll have been a potty equipment expert. Very cool, huh?

The Toilet Chair

Low to the bottom and possible for your child to use by himself. A toilet seat is the starting place for any mother or father looking at toilet training the youngster.

Baby sitting on the potty chair along with his pants down

A toilet chair is actually a small chair that sits on the floor with a recessed area to capture pee and poop. Due to the low elevation, your child can sit back with his foot touching the bottom.

Whenever your baby did his business, you'll be required to bare the articles of the potty seat in to the bin and wash it away in the sink.

Toilet chairs are portable. The capability to take the toilet seat from room to room means that it'll always be close by whenever your toddler has got the urge to visit a toilet.

Advantages

- Can be in virtually any room of the home.

- Childs feet sit comfortably on the floor.

- No great elevation to fall from.

- Easy for your child to take a seat on without your assistance.

Disadvantages

- Cleaning required after every use.

- Still need to teach your child to employ a regular toilet.

- The common seat height is 6 inches, not ideal for a taller toddler.

Various kinds of potty chairs.

You can find different kinds of potty chairs; let us check out each in more details.

- Single piece toilet chair.

- Traditional solitary piece toilet chair.

- Two pieces' toilet chair

- Deluxe toilet chair, etc.

The standard of potty chairs is manufactured out of a single little bit of molded plastic. While this toilet seat will definitely complete the job, this style can be unpleasant to take a seat on and heavy to clean.

Two pieces' toilet chair with removable insert

This is a typical type of modern potty chairs. As the name suggests, this toilet chair comprises of two separate items:

- An outer plastic material seat that helps your child while sitting.

- An inner plastic material bowl that attracts your

baby's waste.

Whenever your baby is completed; simply take away the internal bucket and clean it before coming back it to the toilet chair. Cleaning a detachable insert is a lot easier and quicker than attempting to clean the complete potty chair in the kitchen sink.

Deluxe toilet chair

A deluxe potty seat contains many different great features, including:

- Storage space - Hooks and grab drawers will help you to keep paper or baby wipes close by and ready for use once your child has completed pooping.

- Lights and noises - Whenever your baby has finished his/her business, he/she can press the lever, and it is rewarded with a flushing audio or flashing lighting. Some potty chair even play music whenever your baby rests down.

- Deodorizer - Helps stop your baby's poop from stinking out the home before you get an opportunity to wash the toilet.

- Cushioned chair - Has an incredibly smooth place for your child to do his business.

- Stickers - Some toilet chairs like the My Fun Sticker Toilet feature a group of stickers. These stickers allow your son or daughter to make toilet unique simply for him/her.

- iPad stand - I'm being serious. Some potties include an iPad tablet stand for your child to try out while pooing.

Deluxe potty seats are a capture 22, these features can be extremely useful in getting the child to use the toilet. Around the flipside, each added feature will add mass to the toilet and it is also yet another thing that will require cleaning when it gets covered in pee or poop (an extremely real probability).

Multifunction toilet chair

A multifunction potty seat was created to grow with your child. Below are the various combinations of multifunction toilet chairs:

- 2-in-1 - A toilet seat with a removable toilet seat.

- 3-in-1 - A toilet chair, potty chair and step-stool.

- 4-in-1 - A toilet chair, potty chair, step-stool and storage space compartments

There can be an exemplary case of a 3-in-1 toilet seat; the

Bravo 3-in-1 Toilet, 3-in-1 combination toilet chair.

Personally, I do nothing like a combination of baby equipment. Instead of being great at an individual task they may be average at multiple. Although it may seem inexpensive to buy all-in-one solution; you will put away yourself from stress if you get them separately.

Another downside with mixture potties is they have more parts to them. More items equal more cleaning, and more cleaning equals less quality time with your baby.

Chapter 10

Toilet Chair Features

This section will concentrate on the features you'll need to consider when investing in a potty chair.

Splash guard

Toddler seat with splash safeguard for toilet training boys has the lip of the potty sticks up. This lip is recognized as the splash safeguard and was created to assist with toilet training young males.

If you observe, your little young man won't immediately learn how to position his dangly piece when sitting on the potty, which means that there sometimes will be cases of friendly open fire ending up around your floor.

The splashguard aids in preventing pee from escaping the

potty by bouncing it back to the bowl below, potentially helping you from cleaning pee from the ground.

You might not need a splash guard if you are potty training a woman. Having said that, some girls slightly tilt their pelvis ahead when peeing. This peeing position will begin to see your floor splattered if your toilet chair doesn't have a splash safeguard.

- Stability

The ultimate way to keep the floor clean is by choosing a potty chair that is difficult to tip over. You don't want your son or daughter to lean (or even excitedly leap up to check on her improvement) and also have the toilet seat topple over; sending its material all around the floor.

Two things donate to how easy it really is to spill a toilet:

- Weight - The heavier a toilet is, the harder it'll be to subject upon.

- Foundation of support - The bottom of the toilet sits on your floor. The greater of the bottom that touches the ground, the harder the toilet is to spill.

To check on for stability, place the toilet on to the floor, kneel down before it and put hands left and right of the toilet then apply your bodyweight and change one hand to the other. After evaluating a few, you will begin to have the ability to find a toilet that is a lot harder to suggest than others.

When you have tiles or a wooden floor a plastic lined bottom level is a needed feature. A plastic bottom will stop your toilet from sliding and slipping around your floor while your child attempts to climb aboard.

Chapter 11

How to approach Toilet Training Regression

Is your potty-trained child all of a sudden having incidents? Find out why toilet regression is going on and how to prevent it.

Everything is moving along nicely; your baby appears to have mastered toilet training and also you think you've said goodbye to diapers once and for all. But then, abruptly he begins having mishaps again and you also question what went incorrect. We'll clarify why a kid usually takes a few steps backward as it pertains to toilet training, and how to proceed about it.

Make Certain that It's a genuine Regression

Be confident that a lot of kids experience toilet training regression, it's completely normal. But consider whether your son or daughter was really toilet-trained in the first place. It's very common for periodic setbacks in the first days, weeks, or even many years of toilet training, but understand that a truly toilet trained child should want to be on the toilet. So, a kid that has several incidents every day and doesn't appear to value them shouldn't really be looked as 'toilet trained'. So, consider whether your son or daughter was prepared to toilet teaching; if he was, begin looking for methods of getting back on the right track, if not, speak to your pediatrician about when she/he feels your son or daughter to might prepare yourself.

Don't Overreact

If your son or daughter comes with an accident, don't show disappointment; doing this can make your baby more anxious which, in turn, can result in more toilet problems. Regardless of the frustration you're experiencing, return to diapers because of toilet-training regression, do all you can to remain positive. When you determine if your son or daughter is dried out, clap and cheer if he/she actually is. If he/she is not, just stay non-judgmental and say, "Oops, you'd a major accident, let's go take a seat on the toilet". Be sure you remain upbeat rather than yell at or scold your son or daughter. You want your kids to feel empowered rather than worry that they will be punished if indeed they make a blunder.

Resolve the Main Causes

You're not heading to avoid the setbacks unless you address the precise problem. Make an effort to identify the reason for the regression, as dealing with them can help the child go back to where she was. From the Portion of Developmental and Behavioral Pediatrics at the College or university of Oklahoma Health Sciences Middle and the Director of the kid Study Center. For example, many children start having incidents during times of changeover that may cause stress, such as starting a fresh college or welcoming a fresh sibling. It's likely that, once your lives relax, your son or daughter will master toilet training once more, but even if your son or daughter makes it during the day without mishaps, she still may have mishaps during the night. Many kids aren't dried out at night for a long time once they are dried out throughout the day. Nighttime and naptime control are extremely unique of daytime control. Medical issues can also cause toilet training regression, and constipation is a common one. If a kid has difficulty having a bowel motion, the kid might use the toilet completely to avoid needing to press and strain. Ensure that your child gets enough dietary fiber and a lot of drinking water, but if she's frightened of pooping on the toilet, play video games or read books with her while she rests on the toilet to make it more pleasurable.

Often, accidents happen just because a child is having too much fun playing or doing a task and doesn't want to avoid the performance by going to the toilet. To resolve this example, explain that it's normal to neglect the toilet sometimes and reassure your son or daughter that she's still "a huge lady". Then take her to the toilet every few hours at home and have her teachers to ensure she reaches the toilet frequently. Simple, mild reassurance and reminders to use the toilet will receive a child back again on the right track. Encourage your son or daughter to at least make an effort to use the toilet when she first wakes up, before foods, before bedtime, and immediately before you go out.